Homemade Hand Sanitizer DIY Face Mask

Natural and Effective Hand Sanitizer Recipes, DIY Antibacterial Wipes and Medical Face Masks

D1641509

Olivia Bryant

Content

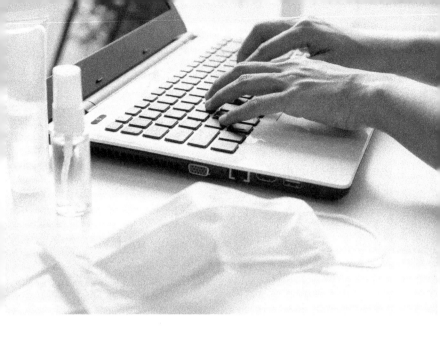

Introduction

Have you ever wondered whether you are safe from infectious diseases like deadly bird flu or rabies? When you are traveling, are you protected from the many infections abroad, from yellow fever to malaria?

Bacteria and viruses are constantly threatening our health, especially if our immunity is weak, because some of them can be spread quickly and cause harsh complications. Of course, considering the age we live in, it's natural that we think of ways to prevent infections, so we can protect ourselves and those who are close to us.

The spread of many viral and bacterial diseases can be prevented by hygienic factors such as efficient sanitation facilities, effective waste disposal, clean water, and of course, personal cleanliness and personal protective equipment (PPE), such as face masks and sanitizers.

But during this time of PPE and personal care product shortages, we all need to use them appropriately so that they are available where they are needed the most - for medical workers and caregivers so that they can take care of you and your loved ones safely.

So, what precautions should you take to stay safe when resources are more limited than ever? How are you supposed to get along without those goods? This book is going to answer these questions and more!

How can you make necessary personal care and personal protection products, such as hand sanitizers, antibacterial wipes, and face masks at home? What works the best against bacteria and viruses? Everything you should know about those topics is here, just flip this page and start to learn!

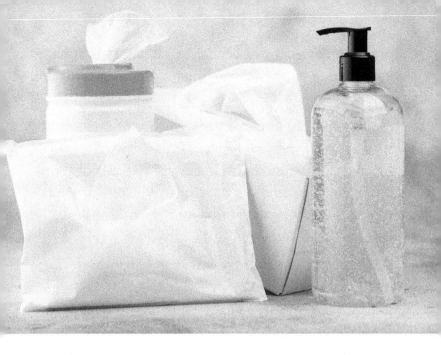

CHAPTER 1. Hand Sanitizers and Antibacterial Wipes

The importance of using hand sanitizers and antibacterial wipes

While handwashing is best for removing germs, hand sanitizers and antibacterial wipes are better than nothing — especially when you don't have access to soap and water. Using a wipe or a hand sanitizer with at least 60 percent alcohol is an important step you should take to avoid getting ill and infecting those around you.

There are essential differences between washing hands with soap and water and cleaning them with sanitizers or wipes. For example, alcohol-based sanitizers don't kill germs, such as the stomach bug called norovirus and some other parasites.

Hand sanitizers also may not get harmful chemicals, such as pesticides and heavy metals like lead off, while handwashing reduces the amount of all types of germs, pesticides, and metals on hands – wipes are more effective, as they can absorb, but still, nothing beats the good old soap and water.

So, knowing when to clean your hands and which method is optimal will give you the best chance of preventing sickness, and the table on the next page is there to show it.

Soap and Water	Hand Sanitizers and Wipes
Before, during, and after preparing food	If water and soap are not available (wash with soap and water as soon as you can.)
Before consuming food	
Before and being in contact with a sick person	
Before and after treating a wound	After touching door handles, elevator buttons, handrails, telephones, etc. in public places
After using the bathroom, cleaning a child who used the bathroom, or changing diapers	
After coughing, sneezing, or blowing your nose	

After touching an animal, animal food, or animal waste
After touching the garbage
If your hands are visibly dirty

** Do **not** use sanitizers, if your hands are visibly greasy or dirty: for example, after playing outdoors, after gardening, or after fishing or camping (unless a handwashing station is not available).*

Portable solutions are the most useful during the peak respiratory virus season because they make it much easier to clean your hands.

It is much more difficult when you sneeze to wash your hands than it is to use a wipe or hand sanitizer, especially when you are outdoors or in a car. Wipes and hand sanitizers are much more convenient, so they make it more likely that people will clean their hands, and that is better than not cleaning at all.

Foam, gel, and liquid sanitizers, their types

Hand sanitizers typically come in foam, gel, or liquid form, and even though it's mostly a matter of personal preference and free choice, there are still some real advantages and disadvantages of both.

Foam sanitizers

A real advantage of foam hand sanitizers is that the product sticks to the hands. It does not slide off the hands as easily as gel sanitizers. This can be very relevant in facilities with waxed floors as sanitizer drips can leave marks on them. Also, when more sanitizer stays on your hands, more hand sanitizer is available to kill the germs on your hands.

A common but misguided "advantage" of foam sanitizers is that "you use less per application, so it's cheaper in the long run", while it's technically true that most foam pumps have a smaller output per push than a gel pump, for a hand sanitizer to be effective, the hands need to stay wet with alcohol for at least 15 seconds. Using less sanitizer per application saves money but drops the effectiveness of the application due to insufficient volume, so this would not be a definite advantage.

Some users of foam sanitizers believe that they are more comfortable to spread around the hands. This is possible because the foam is raised off the skin and can be easily pushed around the hands. However, you hear about the same "advantage" from people who prefer gel, so this is simply a preference.

And their disadvantage is that they are generally more expensive. This is because the foam pumps and ingredients that make the foam sanitizers are rather costly compared to a gel formulation and pump.

Gel sanitizers

Gel sanitizers have been around for decades, and most people seem to understand how to use them. Some people believe that gels are more comfortable to slide in between fingers, around the hands, and to the backs of the hands. Others believe that gels are more convenient to use around fingernails because the gel flows into the cuticles.

The only real disadvantage is that gels easily drip from the hands. Hence sanitizer drips can leave marks on the floor, and less hand sanitizer on the hands means that fewer germs will be killed.

Liquid sanitizers

And liquid sanitizers... they're just liquid sanitizers. Almost like gel, but less dense, so chances that they will drip are even higher.

Drawing the line

To draw the line, there was a study that examined the effect of alcohol-based hand rubs of each format, in doses of 0.7 ml, 1.5 ml, 3 ml. This study found that all forms were less desirable at the higher doses, as they were more challenging to apply than the lower doses. Gels and foams became less clean-feeling, stickier, and slower to dry in higher doses.

Liquids gave a smoother, cleaner, more moisturized feel, but the increased difficulty in applying and handling with the product totally negated these benefits. Overall, the foam and gel formats were more desirable than the liquid. The key desirable properties include fast absorption, soft/moisturized hand feel, not sticky, clean feel, and low smell.

And the conclusion of this study was that the 1.5 ml dose yielded the most acceptable properties with no extreme negative consequences, and the foam provided the benefits of both the gel and liquid combined into a more widely accepted format that may lead to greater hand hygiene compliance.

So, the best hand sanitizer choice between foam, liquid, and gel should depend on which type you will use more often, and one wouldn't be less effective than others, as long as it has at least 60% alcohol or its substitute.

Speaking of alcohol content, the market provides us with two distinct choices: alcohol-based and alcohol-free sanitizers, and both options again have their benefits and drawbacks.

Alcohol-based sanitizers

Alcohol-based products usually contain one of two active ingredients - isopropanol or alcohol. Both are efficient antiseptic products that kill bacteria and germs. The FDA, for maximum efficacy, recommends hand sanitizers contain 60%-95% alcohol.

A common side-effect that is often associated with the constant use of alcohol-based hand sanitizers is the cracking and dryness that it can bring to hands. This occurs because the oils in your skin that retain moisture are being stripped away by alcohol.

The temporary absence of these oils leads to an increase in hand skin irritation. It can even lead to dermatitis symptoms. Another accusation is that the alcohol in these products can damage walls and floors.

Nonetheless, alcohol-based products have been the recommended course of action (second to hand washing) by leading global health organizations such as the FDA, WHO, and the CDC for a long time, and they remain the most used type of sanitizer in health care facilities. Their effectiveness withstands the test of time.

Alcohol-free sanitizers

Most of the alcohol-free products that are available today come in a water-based foam. Those products contain the active ingredient benzalkonium chloride. As opposed to alcohol-based products, most alcohol-free hand sanitizers contain less than 0.1% concentration of benzalkonium, but still provide a comparable level of protection. The rest of the solution is mostly water and will often be filled with skin conditioners such as the extract of green tea and vitamin E.

Typically, these solutions are much gentler on the hands. They also are much less of a threat if ingested accidentally (which is excellent, if you have kids). Alcohol-free hand sanitizers are non-damaging to surfaces and a low fire hazard. One other obvious benefit is their extended protection. Alcohol-based product's bacteria-killing ability ends once the product evaporates, but benzalkonium-based products continue to provide protection long after that.

One possible downside of the alcohol-free solutions is that they most often come in the form of foam, as it requires a special foaming mechanism in the dispenser, even though it usually gives the user a more pleasant experience.

Despite some clear advantages, alcohol-free products have yet to gain recognition in the health market. Alcohol-based gels are still favored by health organizations, which results in them being seen as a more credible solution by the masses.

But both types of products do more or less the same job in killing harmful microbes. Choose the right product by weighing your needs against your environment, budget, and personal preference.

For example, if you work in a school or manufacturing facility, an alcohol-free solution would be the best choice, providing protection from ingestion or fire and peace of mind. But if you work in a hospital that has strict guidelines set by the FDA, you should go with an alcohol-based one.

In terms of budget, alcohol-free sanitizers are less expensive with more applications per gallon. A gallon of each may cost the same, but you will usually get 2,000 to 3,000 more applications out of the foaming hand sanitizers. This is because the dispensing mechanism adds air to the solution during the application, making the product go much further before running out.

Whatever your needs, use an effective hand sanitizer as part of your preventative defense against illness and disease.

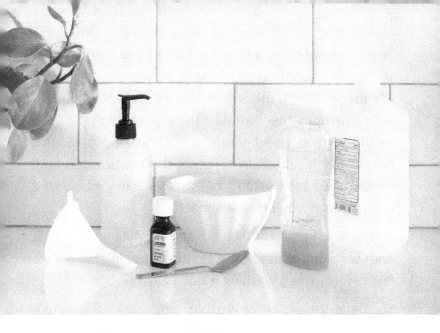

How to make hand sanitizers

As you undoubtedly know, during public health crises bottles of hand sanitizer can sell out really quickly. But don't let that bother you — making your own hand sanitizer is exceptionally easy. DIY sanitizer would even have some advantages compared to store-bought ones, like:

- You can control the ingredients yourself.
- You can customize the smell.
- Within 26 seconds of applying, whatever you put on your body can already be found in your cells! So, it's best to choose good things to put on your skin.

You just have to be a little careful, so you don't mess it up, making sure that all of the tools you use for mixing are pre-sanitized; otherwise, there's a chance that you will corrupt the whole thing. Additionally, it's recommended to let your concoction sit for 72 plus hours after it's done. In doing so, the sanitizer has time to kill any bacteria that might have been introduced during the mixing process in itself.

(Note: To repeat, nothing beats cleaning your hands with soap and water. Hand sanitizer should always be a last resort - when washing is not available.)

So, let's begin with alcohol sanitizers, as they're conventionally the most effective. Again, your sanitizer formulation must have least 60 percent alcohol to be effective, according to the Center of Disease Control and prevention, but it's even better to get above that and aim for at least 75 percent. The best thing to use is a bottle of 99 percent isopropyl alcohol.

Gel Alcohol-Based Hand Sanitizer

The first recipe is really simple, and to make it you'll need:

- Isopropyl alcohol
- Aloe Vera gel
- Tea tree oil
- Gel container
- A common funnel to get your concoction into a bottle.

- Bowl and a whisk to mix it all.

Mix 3 parts isopropyl alcohol to 1 part Aloe Vera gel. Drop a few drips of tea tree oil in to give it a pleasant scent and to align your chakras. Mix everything well, add it to your container, and you're done!

How to use:

- Wipe hands clean of any dirt, if possible
- Apply about a 1.5 ml, nickel-size dose straight to the palm of your hand
- Rub hands, making sure that hand sanitizer gets all over your hands
- Keep going until it is completely absorbed

Liquid Alcohol-Based Spray Hand Sanitizer

The previous aloe mixture gets the job done, but aloe also leaves your skin annoyingly sticky. So, here's a recipe that's less sticky and more potent:

- 1½ cups of isopropyl alcohol
- 2 teaspoons of glycerol
- 1 tablespoon of hydrogen peroxide
- ⅓ cup of distilled water
- Spray container
- A basic funnel to get your concoction into a bottle
- Bowl and a whisk to mix it all together

Combine 1½ cups of isopropyl alcohol with 2 teaspoons of glycerol, add 1 tablespoon of hydrogen peroxide, 2 tablespoons of glycerol, and then pour in ⅓ cup of distilled water. Mix everything well, add it to your container, and you're done!

How to use:

- Wipe hands clean of any dirt, if possible
- Apply about a 1.5 ml, nickel-size dose straight to the palm of your hand
- Rub hands, making sure that hand sanitizer gets all over your hands
- Keep going until it is completely absorbed

Foaming Alcohol-Based Hand Sanitizer

This recipe might be the simplest, yet it's still effective, and to make it you'll need:

- Liquid hand soap
- Isopropyl alcohol
- Foaming container
- A basic funnel to get your concoction into a bottle.
- Bowl and a whisk to mix it all together.

Fill your bottle with ½ centimeter (about ¼ inch) liquid hand soap and fill the rest of the bottle with isopropyl alcohol. You may even need less soap. Foaming hand dispensers vary in how much soap is necessary, so experiment a bit. Mix everything well, add it to your container, and you're done!

How to use:

- Wipe hands clean of any dirt, if possible
- Apply about a 1.5 ml, nickel-size dose straight to the palm of your hand
- Rub hands, making sure that hand sanitizer gets all over your hands
- Keep going until it is completely absorbed

But if you want some alcohol-free options, here's some as well:

Liquid Alcohol-Free Spray Hand Sanitizer

This blend includes essential oils with proven anti-viral and antibacterial properties and adds indispensable Aloe Vera gel for smoothness. Here's what you'll need for this recipe:

- 4 fluid ounce spray bottle, ¾ full of sterile water.
- 1 tablespoon of Aloe Vera gel.
- 10 drops each of cinnamon, clove, rosemary, and eucalyptus essential oils.
- 20 drops of either lemon, orange, or grapefruit essential oil.
- Spray container
- A basic funnel to get your concoction into a bottle.
- Bowl and a whisk to mix it all together

Fill your spray bottle to ¾ with sterile water. Add 1 tablespoon of Aloe Vera gel, 10 drops each of cinnamon, clove, rosemary, and eucalyptus essential oils, then add 20 drops of either lemon, orange, or grapefruit essential oil. Mix everything well, add it to your container, and you're done!

How to use:

- Wipe hands clean of any dirt, if possible
- Apply about a 1.5 ml, nickel-size dose straight to the palm of your hand
- Rub hands, making sure that hand sanitizer gets all over your hands
- Keep going until it is wholly completely

Foaming Alcohol-Free Hand Sanitizer

If you want something foamy – you can use this recipe:

- 3 tablespoons of Aloe Vera gel
- 1 tablespoon of unscented witch hazel
- 15 drops of thieves oil
- 5 drops of lemon oil
- Foaming container
- A basic funnel to get your concoction into a bottle.
- Bowl and a whisk to mix it all together.

Combine 3 tablespoons of Aloe Vera with 1 tablespoon of unscented witch hazel, add 15 drops of thieves oil, then add 5 drops of lemon oil. Mix everything well, add it to your container, and you are done!

How to use:

- Wipe hands clean of any dirt, if possible
- Apply about a 1.5 ml, nickel-size dose straight to the palm of your hand
- Rub hands, making sure that hand sanitizer gets all over your hands
- Keep going until it is completely absorbed

Gel Alcohol-Free Hand Sanitizer

And if you want something similar to the previous one, but in gel form, you can use this recipe:

- Aloe Vera gel
- Witch hazel
- Essential oil – recommended: cinnamon, clove, tea tree
- Gel container
- A basic funnel to get your concoction into a bottle.
- Bowl and a whisk to mix it all together.

Fill your bottle to approximately ⅓ with witch hazel, fill the remaining amount with Aloe Vera gel. For every ounce of your bottle, add 1 or 2 drops of oil, mix everything well, add it to your container, and you are done!

How to use:

- Wipe hands clean of any dirt, if possible

- Apply about a 1.5 ml, nickel-size dose straight to the palm of your hand
- Rub hands, making sure that hand sanitizer gets all over your hands
- Keep going until it is completely absorbed

So, why bother buying hand soap and hand sanitizer when you can easily make your own for very little? Don't answer—rhetorical question!

Dry and wet antibacterial wipes, their types

It is common for people to believe that regular cleaning with soap and water is enough to protect the skin. However, some studies have shown that soap can also be drying and cause irritation.

Frequent contact with water and soap strips the natural oils from the skin whereas wet wipes can gently dissolve irritants while helping maintain the skin's natural PH. Wet wipes are pre-moistened with a formula to cleanse, restore, and protect skin with just a single wipe.

Modern wet wipes have played an important role in preventing contamination and transmission of infectious diseases. They can be used to cleanse, moisturize, and deodorize, and offer antibacterial and barrier protection.

Key benefits of using wet wipes are:

- They are perfectly PH Balanced
- Most of them are enriched with aloe and a light scent to soothe the skin and reduce odors
- They leave the skin soft and clean
- They are ideal when running water is unavailable
- Improved skin health
- They allow for quick and easy hygiene throughout the day
- They are suitable for frequent use
- They raise personal hygiene standards
- They prevent the development of Dermatitis

But there are actually dry wipes too! These can serve as a time-saving solution for ensuring adequate cleansing and skincare are carried out. Dry wipes are manufactured with a dry texture without any added cleaning solutions and are ideal for use as a replacement for your usual washcloth or sponge.

Both dry and wet antibacterial wipes can be categorized into: sanitizing and disinfecting.

Disinfecting kills germs on surfaces or objects, purifying works by using chemicals to kill bacteria. This process is mostly not about cleaning dirty surfaces, it is more about killing germs on a surface, and it lowers the risk of infection spreading drastically.

Sanitizing is softer than disinfecting. It lowers the number of germs on surfaces and objects to a safe level, set by public health requirements or standards. This process works by cleaning surfaces or objects, slowing the infection spread.

Sanitizing Wipes

Sanitizing wipes are used to kill germs and bacteria on the hands when handwashing is not possible. They can remove dirt and sweat before they settle into your pores, and some no-rinse wipes can even remove waterproof makeup.

These are usually pre-moistened and come either individually packaged or in one larger container that can be resealed.

And these, in their turn, also have three main types:

- Hand-sanitizing wipes that are used to kill germs and bacteria from the hands when handwashing is not possible.
- Face cleansing wipes that are used to remove the oil and dirt from the face. They help to remove makeup as well.
- Baby wipes that are the most common type of sanitizing wipes since they are designed to be used on babies and infants who have very sensitive skin.

Disinfecting wipes

Disinfecting wipes provide a lot of daily benefits when used at home. You can take advantage of these as they help to make housecleaning faster and more efficient. For one, wipes can be used in the kitchen when cleaning kitchen appliances, kitchen utensils, or just the table. They can also be used to clean children's playrooms and in the bedroom to clean dirty surfaces and to avoid the spread of germs and diseases.

Disinfecting wipes are amazingly helpful in cleaning and disinfecting doorknobs, toilet seats, and bathroom counters.

They are actually the best at cleaning the bathroom. The bathroom is typically the dirtiest place in the house, as it is often filled with germs, bacteria, and viruses. Germs can quickly spread to surfaces if you use cleaning cloths and sponges, so it is still best to utilize medical-grade disinfecting wipes when dealing with it.

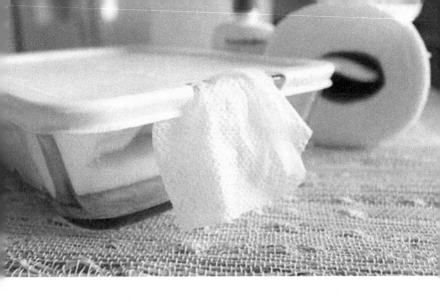

How to make antibacterial wipes

Can't find proper sanitizing or disinfecting wipes in stores? Not only is it easy to make your own at home, but they're cheap, effective, and infinitely usable too!

Sanitizing wipes

It's really easy to make your own sanitizing hand wipes at home using just a few ingredients that you may already have. The main ingredient featured here is isopropyl (rubbing) alcohol. Isopropyl alcohol denatures the protective outer proteins of microbes by dissolving their membranes to kill germs and bacteria quickly, and this is what it is known and used for.

Things that you'll need:

- ¼ cup of isopropyl alcohol, 60% or above
- ¼ cup of distilled water

- 1 tablespoon of hydrogen peroxide
- 1 teaspoon of glycerin
- 30 paper towels cut in half
- Glass, stainless steel, or plastic container for storage
- Bowl and a whisk to mix it all together.

Put all of the ingredients in a bowl, use a whisk to mix them together really well. Stack the paper towels in a storage container, pour the liquid mixture over the paper towels, and then close the container and shake it well. Make sure all of the paper towels are soaked thoroughly.

How to use sanitizing hand wipes:

- Shake the container before each use, wring out the wipe if needed.
- Wipe hands all over and let them air dry.

Disinfecting wipes

Many homemade cleaning wipes are great for removing dirt, but they're not proper disinfectants. Most DIY cleaning wipes only use vinegar, Castile soap, or detergents like Sal Suds or natural dish soap. While those types of ingredients are great for making homemade cleaning wipes, they are not effective disinfectants.

To make effective homemade disinfecting wipes, the liquid disinfecting solution needs to be at least 70% alcohol.

It's easy to make DIY disinfecting wipes that are natural and don't have any harsh chemicals. You just need the right recipe. And here it is:

- 3 cups of 70%+ isopropyl alcohol
- ¾ teaspoon of hydrogen peroxide (3% hydrogen peroxide)
- 20 drops of lemon essential oil
- 15 drops of clove essential oil
- 10 drops of cinnamon bark essential oil
- 5 drops of eucalyptus radiata essential oil
- 5 drops of rosemary essential oil
- Glass, stainless steel, or plastic container for storage
- Bowl and a whisk to mix it all together.

Put all of ingredients in a bowl, use a whisk to mix them together really well. Stack the paper towels in a storage container, pour the liquid mixture over the paper towels, and then close the container and shake it well. Make sure all of the paper towels are soaked thoroughly.

How to use these wipes to clean surfaces:

- Shake the container well before each use.
- If the surface is visibly dirty, pre-clean the surface with an all-purpose cleaner or cleaning wipes
- Pull a wipe out of the container, making sure that the wipe is wet with a disinfecting solution.

- Wipe hard, non-porous surfaces with the wipe until the surface is visibly wet.
- Leave the wet surface for a few minutes and allow to air dry.

*Do **not** use disinfectant wipes on your skin, because they may cause skin and eye irritation. Disinfectant wipes are not intended for use on humans or animals. Disinfectant wipes are designed for use on hard, non-porous surfaces.*

How & when to use a hand sanitizer and antibacterial wipes effectively, safety concerns

As with other household products, the key here is proper storage and usage.

So, make sure to:

- Always read and always follow instructions on all products before using them.
- In case of eye contact, rinse with water.
- If inflammation or redness develops, ask a doctor.
- Keep away from fire or flame.
- When not in use, store the product correctly in a safe place out of the reach of children.
- Avoid contact with the face, eyes, and broken skin.

And when using sanitizer:

- Use one or two squirts or pumps of the product.
- Rub hands together briskly, including the front and back, between fingers, around and under nails until hands are dry.

Or when using wipes:

- Wipe all areas of hands until they are visibly clean.
- Use one or more wipes and dispose of them in an appropriate trash container.

- Let hands air dry.

Always remember that using hand sanitizing products frequently can make your hands very dry.

There's that one step we all tend to forget about after washing our hands or applying hand sanitizer – that vital layer of hand lotion. Ironically, we can develop dry cracks in the skin by over-washing it, giving bacteria an entry point into our bodies.

But why is handwashing so harsh on our skin?

The outer layer of our skin is composed of wax and oils, and it acts both as a guard that maintains natural moisture inside and the shield from the outside. Suds created by soaps and sanitizers can break down this natural barrier.

Not applying hand cream can lead to dryness, redness, itching, flaking, discomfort, and in severe cases, cracks in the skin. Those with preexisting dermatologic conditions like eczema can experience worsening symptoms.

How should we clean our hands to avoid skin dryness?

After you have used the cleaning product and your hands are dry, apply moisturizer all over your hands, paying particular attention to where they may be prone to cracking. You don't need fancy formulas with specialty additives or lotions made for hospital wash stations, which are made to be compatible with disinfectant, standard hand cream is enough.

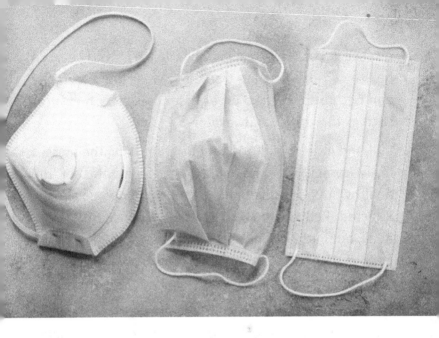

CHAPTER 2. Face Masks

The importance of wearing face mask

Facemasks help to limit the spread of germs. When someone coughs, sneezes, or talks, they may release tiny drops into the air that can infect others. If someone is ill, face masks reduce the number of germs that the wearer releases, protecting other people from becoming sick. And if someone is not ill, the face mask also protects the wearer's nose and mouth from splashes or sprays of body fluids.

Both surgical masks and respirators have been shown to prevent various respiratory infections in health care workers, but masks might work better at preventing disease in hospitals than in public. In part this is because health care workers are trained to wear them correctly and because they take other essential safety measures such as thorough handwashing.

Still, the most significant benefit of masking the masses likely comes not from shielding the mouths of the healthy but from covering the mouths of people already infected. People who feel ill aren't supposed to go out at all, but initial evidence suggests that sometimes even people without symptoms may also transmit viruses without knowing they're infected.

Data from contact-tracing efforts—in which researchers monitor the health of people who recently interacted with someone confirmed to have an infection—suggest nearly half of transmissions occur before the infected person shows symptoms. And some seem to contract and clear the virus without ever feeling sick.

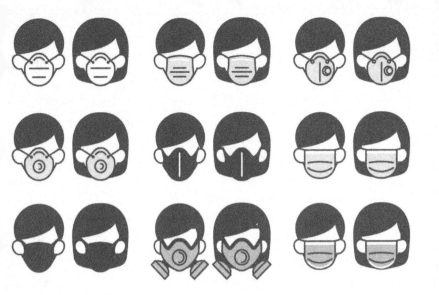

Types of face masks

As mentioned previously, there are 2 main types of masks that are used to prevent respiratory infections: respirators and surgical masks, sometimes referred to as medical or face masks. These two types differ by the type and size of infectious particles they are able to filter.

Surgical masks

Surgical masks are loose-fitting face masks that cover your mouth, chin, and nose. They're typically used to:

- Protect the wearer from large particle droplets
- Prevent the spread of infectious respiratory secretions from the wearer to others

Surgical masks vary in design, but the mask itself is commonly flat and rectangular with folds or pleats. Top of the mask has a soft metal strip that can be formed to your nose. Masks can come in different thicknesses and with varying protecting abilities. These properties may also affect how easily it is for you to breathe through the mask.

Long straight ties or elastic bands help hold a medical mask in the right place on your face. These can either be tied behind your head or looped over your ears. If worn correctly, it blocks the most of large-particle droplets, sprays, splashes, or splatter that may contain germs (viruses and bacteria), keeping them from reaching your mouth and nose.

Respirator masks

A respirator is a more tight-fitting face mask that covers your mouth, chin, and nose. In addition to sprays, splashes, and large droplets, it can also filter out 95 percent of different microscopic particles. This percentage includes bacteria and viruses.

The respirator generally comes in oval or circular shapes, and it is designed to fit your face firmly with elastic bands, forming a tight seal. Some respirators may have an attachment called "exhalation valve," which can help with breathing and the buildup of heat and humidity.

Respirators aren't one-size-fits-all, they must be fit-tested before use to be sure that a right seal is formed because you won't receive the appropriate protection if the mask doesn't seal to your face well.

After being fit-tested the first time, users of respirators must continue to do a seal check each and every time they put one on. It's also important to note that the right seal is rarely achieved in some groups, including children and people with facial hair.

How to make face masks

Because of the urgent need for face masks, many people have begun making their own from various materials, such as antimicrobial pillowcases and scarfs. The Center of Disease Control indicates that in settings where medical face masks are unavailable, homemade face masks can be used as a last resort, and they're definitely better than nothing.

The best fabric for homemade masks is a tightly woven, 100% cotton fabric. Things like denim, bedsheets, and heavyweight shirts are all excellent options.

Layers are crucial to making an effective mask. It's also important that the mask forms a snug seal over the mouth and nose so that particles can't get in through the gaps.

Masks with a silky outer layer, a middle layer of a thick, tightly woven material like nylon or cotton, and then comfortable cotton on the inside are ideal. Avoid knit fabrics (e.g., jersey t-shirts) because they create holes when they stretch, which the viruses could get through.

Make sure to prewash fabrics using hot water to kill germs and to pre-shrink the material, so it doesn't change shape.

So, how do you make a DIY face mask?

Materials:

- Fabric such as a microfiber cloth, washcloth, or just cotton.
- Elastic bands or hair ties
- Scissors or a sharp knife
- Sewing machine or threads and needle

Steps:

- Start with two rectangles of fabric, 11 inches by 5 inches (or 12 inches by 6 inches for a bigger head).
- Sew the layers together, then sew the bottom edge closed.
- Fold over one side edge and start sewing the fabric so that the elastic band or hair tie is inside the fold.
- Once you've started it, pull the elastic taut and sew down the rest of the fold.
- Repeat on the other side.
- Be sure to backstitch (sew over multiple times) at the beginning and end of the seam, since the elastic will be pulling at those spots.

This is as simple as it gets, so you can make many of these, spending minimal time, effort, and resources.

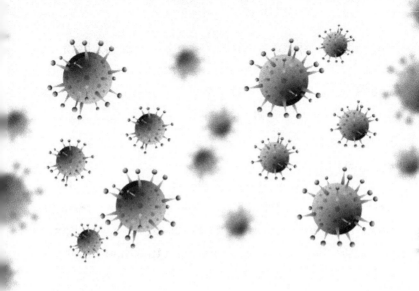

CHAPTER 3. Bacteria and Viruses

The difference between bacteria and virus

Bacteria and viruses are the most common causes of human diseases. When you, for example, shake hands, touch a surface, or are exposed to someone's sneeze droplets, you come into contact with bacteria and viruses, which can enter the body when you touch your mouth, nose, or eyes.

But even though both bacteria and viruses can cause mild to severe infections, they are very different. It's important to understand that difference because bacterial and viral infections must be treated differently.

So, a bacterium is a single but complex cell that can survive on its own, inside or outside the body. They multiply by splitting in half, and some of them can unbelievably double their numbers once in 20 minutes. That's why, even though they are small, bacteria can impact our health significantly.

Humans bear trillions and trillions of bacteria outside and inside our bodies, and most of them keep us healthy by supporting functions like digestion. They gain energy from the same essential sources as humans, including proteins, sugars, and fats. Some bacteria have adapted to live within human or animal hosts, while others live and multiply in the environment.

Viruses are not cells. They are much smaller than any cell. In fact, viruses are fundamentally just capsules with genetic material. Viruses are not like any other group of infectious microorganisms because they are the only group that is unable to replicate beyond the host cell. Because viruses do not eat food like bacteria - instead, they seize materials and energy straight from the host cells.

And viruses are known to infect almost every type of organisms and microorganisms on earth. Some viruses, called bacteriophages, can even infect bacteria.

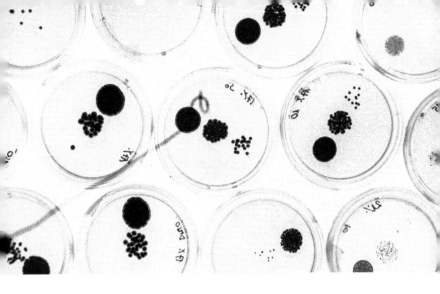

Bacterial and viral infections

And as the names suggest, bacteria cause bacterial infections, and viruses cause viral infections.

And there's an essential difference between what we call infection and disease. Infection, often the first step, happens when bacteria, viruses, or other microbes that cause disease to enter your body and begin to multiply. The disease occurs when the cells of your body get damaged — succeeding the infection — and signs of an illness appear.

Once the virus manages to get inside your body, it attacks healthy cells, taking them over to reproduce and spread throughout your body. Viruses transfer from one host to another by sneezes, coughs, vomits, bites from infected insects or animals, exposure to infected bodily fluids through activities such as sexual intercourse, or sharing hypodermic needles. To grow their number, viruses attack cells in your body, highjacking the processes that make cells work. Most of the time, host cells are eventually destroyed.

Viruses are guilty of causing many diseases, including:

- Aids
- Common cold
- Ebola virus
- Genital herpes
- Influenza
- Measles
- Chickenpox and shingles

Whereas bacteria-caused infections are commonly restricted to one area of the body — like an ear infection or strep throat — viral infections tend to spread more quickly and affect the whole body. Many disease-causing bacteria produce toxins — powerful chemicals that damage cells and make you ill.

Other bacteria can directly invade and damage tissues. To lead to disease, pathogenic bacteria must gain access to the body through contaminated food or water, cuts, breathing in the exhaled droplets when an infected person coughs or sneezes, close contact with an infected person, contact with the feces of an infected person, or indirectly, by touching contaminated surfaces – such as toilet handles, taps, toys, and nappies.

Examples of bacterial infections include:

- Whooping cough
- Strep throat

- Ear infection
- Urinary tract infection
- Mild skin irritation
- Lethal pneumonia

It can be challenging to tell exactly what causes a disease because viral and bacterial infections can bring similar symptoms. Your doctor may request a sample of your stool, urine, and blood for a 'culture' test to have the bugs identified under a microscope.

What works the best against bacterial infections

Bacterial infections range from severe to mild, and some may even be deadly life-threatening. They can affect your blood, your skin, an organ in your body, or your entire gastrointestinal tract.

The number of people who acquire antibiotic-resistant bacteria grows each year, and the number of deaths from these infections is also increasing. Therefore, it is genuinely vital to learn how to prevent bacterial infections.

Proper handwashing is first in the list of the best ways to prevent both bacterial and viral infections. But although hand washing is effective and straightforward, it is often overlooked. Other great methods of avoiding infection include protecting your nose and mouth when you cough or sneeze, avoiding touching your mouth, nose, and eyes, cleaning and disinfecting counters and all other kitchen surfaces, cooking foods using proper temperatures and techniques, refrigerating foods promptly, following doctor's orders regarding immunizations and vaccinations, using antibiotics appropriately, practicing good hygiene around pets, and avoiding contact with wild animals.

What works the best against viral infections

What works the best against viral infections is similar to what works the best against bacterial infections.

People can prevent or help to prevent many of the viral infections by commonsense measures to protect themselves and others. Frequently and wholly cleaning your hands with soap and sanitizers, consuming only liquids and foods that have been appropriately treated or prepared, avoiding contact with contaminated surfaces and infected people, coughing and sneezing into tissues or into the upper arm, using safe sex practices, preventing bites by mosquitoes, ticks, and other arthropods – it all helps.

Immune globulins and vaccines can help the body to defend itself against diseases caused by certain viruses better. Good vaccines can even totally eradicate viral diseases. Smallpox was eliminated recently, in 1978. Polio has been eradicated with the exception of just a few countries where religious sentiment and logistics interfere with the practices of vaccination. Measles has been almost fully eradicated from some parts of the world, such as the Americas.

So, the right precautionary measures are scarier to bacteria and viruses than they are to us.

Conclusion

I sincerely appreciate your purchase of this book that reveals useful information about everything you need to know about Homemade Hand Sanitizers, Antibacterial Wipes, and Face Masks. I hope you love it.

If you would like to leave a comment, you can do it at the Order section->Digital orders, in your account.

Stay safe and healthy!

CPSIA information can be obtained
at www.ICGtesting.com
Printed in the USA
BVHW040957150720
583786BV00007B/138